Simple Cheat Sheet for Romantic Sex

15 Tips for Couples to Make Sex More Romantic and Intimate

Cheryl Bach

Simple Cheat Sheet for Romantic Sex

©2024 by Cheryl Bach

All rights reserved. No part of this publication may be reproduced, distributed, or transmitted in any form or by any means, including photocopying, recording, or other electronic or mechanical methods, without the prior written permission of the publisher, except in the case of brief quotations embodied in critical reviews and certain other noncommercial uses permitted by copyright law. For permission requests, write to the publisher at the address below.

Publisher: IntimateInk Press

Email: intimateinkpress@gmail.com

This book is a work of nonfiction intended for informational purposes only. The content of this book is based on the author's research, knowledge, and experience, and it is provided with the understanding that the author and publisher are not engaged in rendering legal, medical, or professional advice. The information in this book is not a substitute for professional guidance or assistance. Readers should consult with relevant professionals for advice and assistance regarding their specific situations. The author and publisher disclaim any liability for any loss or risk, personal or otherwise, which is incurred as a consequence, directly or indirectly, of the use and application of any of the contents of this book.

Cover design by IntimateInk Press

Interior layout and design by IntimateInk Press

Printed in USA

Fonts: Google fonts

Image: Freepik.com. This cover has been designed using assets from Freepik.com

For permission to use copyrighted material from this book, please contact the copyright holder listed above.

First Edition: 2024

Distributed by Amazon.com, Inc.

Cheryl Bach

Table of Contents

Cheryl Bach

Introduction

Welcome to Simple Cheat Sheet for Romantic Sex: 15 Tips for Couples to Make Sex More Romantic and Intimate, a book that presents a comprehensive guide for couples looking to deepen their bond and spice up their lives in the bedroom. Sex is an essential part of any romantic relationship, yet many couples find themselves falling into patterns that are predictable, repetitive, or unfulfilling. This book offers a simple and practical solution that can transform your sexual experience with your partner from mediocre to magical.

The idea behind this book is to provide couples with an easy-to-follow guide that outlines the most effective and proven approaches to increase intimacy and maintain a level of excitement while making love. Drawing on years of research and consultation from expert sex therapists, we have distilled the 15 most important tips that can help couples enjoy more romantic and intimate sex.

Whether you're in a long-term relationship or just starting out, the tips presented in this book are designed to help you and your partner explore and connect in new ways. From creating a more intimate environment to exploring new positions and techniques, each chapter takes a deep dive into a different aspect of romantic sex. Additionally, we have included tips on how to communicate your desires and boundaries effectively and, most importantly, how to prioritize your partner's needs and desires in an intimate setting.

Throughout the book, we emphasize the importance of communication, trust, and safety in maintaining intimacy. We discuss how physical touch can help create a more powerful emotional connection. We also delve into the many ways that engaged communication before, during, and after sexual encounters can contribute to feelings of closeness and connectedness.

Our goal with Simple Cheat Sheet for Romantic Sex: 15 Tips for Couples to Make Sex More Romantic and Intimate is to provide a practical and easy-to-follow guide that can help couples create a more fulfilling and loving sexual relationship. The tips included in this book are designed to be applicable to any couple, regardless of experience level, age, or background.

We hope that this guide will serve as a valuable resource for couples seeking to explore and enhance their intimacy in the bedroom. So sit back, relax, and get ready to embark on a journey toward a more satisfying and deeply connected sexual relationship with your partner.

Simple Cheat Sheet for Romantic Sex

Chapter 1

Set the Mood

When it comes to romance, creating the right ambiance goes a long way. A romantic atmosphere can help create feelings of intimacy and facilitate a deeper connection between partners. Setting the mood might seem trivial in the grand scheme of sexual encounters, but it can make a significant impact on making your sexual experiences with your partner more memorable and satisfying.

So, how can you create the perfect setting?

Firstly, set up the room to be conducive for intimacy. Remove any distractions such as phones and electronics that may interrupt the good vibes. Invest in some scented candles for a soft and lovely ambiance. The flicking glow of candles creates a warm and cozy environment and can help enhance intimacy between partners.

Choose a scent that both you and your partner enjoy. Make sure the candle wax is natural and free from harmful chemicals that can affect the quality of the air. Scents such as lavender, vanilla, and jasmine can help promote relaxation and reduce stress, helping couples feel more at ease with each other.

In addition to candles, consider adding some soft lighting to the room. Choose lamps, dimmer switches, or fairy lights to create a warm and inviting atmosphere. Soft, ambient lighting can help partners feel relaxed and let their guard down. Ensure there is enough light to see each other but not too much that it ruins the mood.

Lastly, set the tone with some music. Music can help drown out any background noise and create a relaxing atmosphere while setting the rhythm. Build a playlist of songs you both enjoy beforehand, so there's no need to fiddle with your phone later. Invest in a high-quality Bluetooth speaker or sound system to ensure the music is clear and loud enough to enjoy without being overwhelming.

Why is it a top tip for couples to make sex more romantic and intimate?

Creating a romantic atmosphere is essential because it helps partners relax, drop their defenses and create a pleasant environment. A relaxed partner is more likely to be aroused and receptive to the pleasure experience. It also helps partners feel more comfortable with each other, which enhances intimacy and promotes stronger connections.

In conclusion, creating a romantic atmosphere using candles, music, and dim lights is an effective way to enhance intimacy, establish closeness, and enjoy a more satisfying sexual experience with your partner. Embrace the idea of taking the time to create the right ambiance, and you'll be amazed at how quickly your sexual experiences become more passionate and loving.

Chapter 2

Focus on Each Other

In today's age of rapid communication and constant technology bombardment, it can be difficult to disconnect and focus on just one thing at a time. However, when it comes to intimate moments, focusing entirely on your partner is crucial. Removing all types of distractions, including phones, TVs and other devices, helps establish an intimate connection with your partner.

To prioritize your partner, start by switching off or silencing your phones and electronic devices before sex. Get rid of any personal items that may distract you and ruin the moment with your partner.

Simple Cheat Sheet for Romantic Sex

Next, create an environment that promotes intimacy. A bedroom should be well-kept, organized, and comfortable. Choose lighting that isn't too bright, use soft throws and pillows, and put on some relaxing music in the background.

Once you both are comfortable, focus solely on your partner and the moment. Be present with each other, listen to what they're saying, observe how they're responding, and take in every bit of pleasure and intimacy you can get. Pay attention to both verbal and non-verbal communication, responding accordingly.

You can also take the time to explore each other's interests and desires. Engaging in conversation about each other's preferences and fantasies can help create a more intimate bond. Setting the right mood and removing distractions is equally important in this regard.

Why is it a top tip for couples looking to make sex more Romantic and Intimate?

Removing distractions and focusing entirely on your partner enhances intimacy and boosts emotional connection. Sex is more than a physical act; it requires an emotional connection, spontaneity, and vulnerability that requires focus and commitment. Creating a romantic connection requires trust and emotional connection, which can only be achieved by removing all distractions and focusing on your partner.

Focusing on each other leads to a deeper, more profound connection. It lays the foundation for positive communication and physical touch, which is vital to sexual experiences. Moreover, when both partners are focused on each other, they can provide each other with positive feedback, which will make the experience even more satisfying.

In conclusion, focusing on each other by removing distractions such as phones or TVs is an essential tip that can take your intimacy with your partner to the next level. Focusing on your partner helps you create a deeper connection, boost emotional ties and enjoy more meaningful sexual experiences. By committing to paying attention to your partner during sex, you'll find that the experience becomes more enjoyable, fulfilling and intimate.

Chapter 3

Take it Slow

In today's fast-paced lifestyle, taking things slow can seem counterintuitive. However, when it comes to having a romantic and intimate sexual experience, slowing things down is a crucial tip that often gets overlooked. Slowing things down entails taking time to savor each moment, enjoy each other's touch, and prolong pleasure.

To put this tip into practice, start by setting aside enough time for intimacy with your partner that you both feel comfortable with. Do not rush things. Taking the time to build anticipation and allowing your sexual energy to slowly build up can be incredibly exhilarating. Engage in sensual activities like soft touching, eye contact, and deep breathing before any physical contact has begun.

Simple Cheat Sheet for Romantic Sex

When touching, let your fingers glide over your partner's body, exploring and discovering one another's erogenous zones. There is no need to be in a hurry; take your time and enjoy every inch of your partner's body. Use soft, slow touches to help create an atmosphere of relaxation and sensuality. Pay attention to your partner's reactions and take cues from them to explore areas that ignite sensations.

As things begin to heat up, the pace can indeed pick up, but there's still a great deal of room to enjoy a slower, more sensual pace. Instead of rushing straight to intercourse, take the time to engage in other forms of intimacy. You may want to explore each other through kissing, caressing, or exploring one another's various erogenous zones.

Why is it a top tip for couples looking to make sex more Romantic and Intimate?

Slowing things down provides you with time to focus on each other's enjoyment, which fosters intimacy and helps to create a more profound emotional connection. When you slow things down, you have the chance to explore each other's preferences and turn-ons. This enables you to learn your partner's likes and dislikes, leading to a better understanding of their overall sexual needs.

Taking it slow also allows you to prolong pleasure, developing a more profound and satisfying experience. It helps to bring both partners to a heightened state of arousal. Taking the time to focus on each other's pleasure can lead to a more intense, passionate, and loving sexual connection.

Slowing things down is particularly essential for couples who may have been together for a long time. In many cases, sex can become routine, with little attention paid to each other's pleasure and desires. By slowing things down, couples can rediscover one another's sexual interests and build excitement.

In conclusion, taking things slow is an indispensable tip for couples who want to make sex more romantic and intimate. It encourages partners to slow down and savor every moment of the experience, focusing on each other's pleasure and building up anticipation for a more fulfilling experience. It enables couples to rediscover each other's sexual preferences and desires, promoting a more profound emotional connection.

Slowing things down may sound counterintuitive but is a highly effective way to develop a deeper, more satisfying, and enjoyable experience. It's an essential component of any intimate relationship and should be embraced by couples looking for a more romantic and intimate sexual experience. Remember, the goal is not to rush through the process but to take your time and enjoy every bit of pleasure and intimacy that you can get. By practicing this tip, you can create a more profound emotional and physical connection with your partner and enjoy fulfilling and engaging sexual experiences.

Simple Cheat Sheet for Romantic Sex

Chapter 4

Use Your Senses

When it comes to having a romantic and intimate sexual experience, engaging all five senses is an important and often overlooked tip. Engaging all five senses helps create a multisensory experience, making the encounter more memorable and meaningful.

Here are a few tips on how to engage all five senses to make sex more romantic and intimate:

Sight: Creating visual appeal can be as simple as lighting candles, setting the mood with soft lighting or creating a romantic atmosphere. The way you dress and how you present yourself can also be visually appealing. You can also create a visual appeal by using a mirror, which can add to the excitement by allowing you and your partner to watch each other, thus increasing the level of intimacy.

Sound: Including sound involves being more vocal and communicating with your partner during the experience. Verbally expressing your pleasure or telling your partner what you want can help to build a deeper connection between partners. The sounds that fill the room can also add to the sensory experience. You could play soft music or choose to leave some natural background noise to create a soothing environment where you can enjoy sex.

Taste: Engaging the sense of taste can involve all kinds of methods, including using edible treats such as whipped cream, chocolate, or strawberries on one another's body. You could also use flavored lubricants. Also, using your partner's taste to explore their erogenous zones can be an exciting and sensual way to increase the intimacy of the moment.

Touch: Using touch is undoubtedly one of the most crucial ways to make sex more romantic and intimate. Touching during sex involves exploring every inch of your partner's body with your hands, lips, and other sensitive parts of your body. Your touch needs to be delicate, soft, and slow, caressing every part of your lover's body. Touch encourages intimacy and creates a powerful bond between you and your partner. Use different fabrics such as silk or satin to incorporate the sense of touch into your romantic experience.

Smell: Incorporating different scents into your sexual experience can turn up the heat and make the moment more romantic. You may try using scented candles, massage oils, or even a perfumed room spray. The scent that you choose will help set the tone for the rest of the experience and can positively impact the overall mood.

Simple Cheat Sheet for Romantic Sex

Engaging all five senses can make a significant difference in the level of intimacy during sex. It transports you away from everyday reality and provides a multi-dimensional experience that is rich and satisfying. The senses work together to create a holistic and profound emotional connection with your partner. By using different methods, such as soft lighting, scents, taste, touch, and sound, you can heighten the intensity of the experience.

The use of all five senses in our sexual experiences is what makes this tip one of the top tips for couples to make sex more romantic and intimate. Engaging all five senses requires attention, focus, and intentionality from both partners. It helps create a deeper level of communication and understanding between partners.

When we engage all the senses, we promote vulnerability and openness with our partner, which in turn can lead to a better connection and increased intimacy. Also, when we stimulate our senses during sex, we trigger feel-good hormones in the brain, such as dopamine, oxytocin, and serotonin that help us feel more pleasure and intimacy.

One important thing to keep in mind is that engaging all the senses is entirely dependent on your preference as a couple. The possibilities are endless, and you should choose what works best for both of you. Experiment with different methods and find what works best for both of you.

In conclusion, engaging all five senses during sex is an effective way to make it more romantic and intimate. Experimenting with different methods to enhance sight, sound, taste, touch, and smell will result in a more profound emotional connection with your partner, create a multisensory experience, and produce feel-good hormones in the brain, thus improving the level of pleasure and intimacy. Couples who incorporate this tip are often more relaxed, playful, and feel freer in their relationship, enjoying a more fulfilled sexual experience.

Chapter 5

Practice Mindfulness

Are you ever in the middle of a sexual experience, but your mind is lingering on other things such as work, bills, or even what you are going to do next? Worrying about these things takes away from the experience and can cause you to miss out on the deep emotional connection that can be formed during sex. By practicing mindfulness, you can be fully present and engaged during the experience, and it can help to deepen the intimacy between you and your partner.

Here are a few tips on how to practice mindfulness during sex:

Breathe: Focusing on your breath can help you stay grounded and present in the moment. Take deep inhales and exhales, and sync your breathing with your partner's; this will help both of you relax and enter a state of heightened awareness.

Focus on sensations: Direct your attention to the physical sensations of the moment. Feel the touch of your partner's hands, the warmth of their breath on your skin, and the sensation of each movement. Allow yourself to become immersed in these sensations, and let go of any racing thoughts.

Let go of expectations: It's important to avoid having any expectations about how the experience is supposed to unfold. Allow it to be different every time and be open to new possibilities. Be curious and explore with your partner to find new things that turn you both on.

Slow down: Our minds are often running at full speed, and we rush through sexual experiences. By slowing down and taking your time, you can become more present and mindful of the moment. Enjoy the entire experience, from foreplay to post-coital cuddling.

Use all your senses: Consider engaging all your senses to stay present in the moment. Take in the scent of your partner's skin, listen to the sounds of their breathing and moans, appreciate the view of their body, taste them, and feel the touch of their skin.

Practicing mindfulness during sex is a powerful way to deepen intimacy and make sex more romantic. When you're present in the moment and fully engaged with your partner, you create a deeper emotional bond, which can lead to a highly satisfying experience for both of you. By focusing on the sensations of the experience and letting go of any expectations, you can fully immerse yourself in the moment and enjoy everything the experience has to offer.

Simple Cheat Sheet for Romantic Sex

The reason why mindfulness is one of the top tips for couples to make sex more romantic and intimate is due to the fact that it helps to create a more present and genuine emotional connection between partners. It's easy to get lost in our thoughts during sex, but being mindful helps us stay grounded and connected with our partner. By being fully present and aware of the physical sensations of the moment, we can deepen the intimacy within the relationship.

Moreover, mindfulness helps individuals let go of any anxious or negative thoughts they might have during sex, improving the overall experience. It improves the concentration and focus on the present moment. When couples are fully present and engaged with each other, it helps to build trust and respect and promote more fulfilling sexual experiences.

Incorporating mindfulness techniques can also help couples navigate difficult emotional states such as jealousy, guilt, or shame surrounding the experience. Name it to tame it. Acknowledging these emotions and working through them together can create a deeper understanding and connection between partners.

In summary, practicing mindfulness is an essential tip for couples to make sex more romantic and intimate. By focusing on the present moment and physical sensations, letting go of expectations and preconceived notions, and using all the senses, partners can create a deeper emotional connection during sex. Mindfulness also helps to build trust and respect within the relationship and navigate difficult emotions that may arise. So if you want to experience a more meaningful and satisfying sexual experience with your partner, try incorporating mindfulness practices into your routine.

Chapter 6

Share Deep Emotions

Sex can be an incredibly intimate and emotional experience, and it's essential to create a safe space where both partners feel comfortable expressing their deepest thoughts, desires, and feelings. Sharing deep emotions during sex can deepen intimacy, trust, and communication within the relationship and lead to more fulfilling experiences.

Here are a few tips on how to go about sharing deep emotions during sex:

Build trust: Before opening up emotionally, it's essential to build trust with your partner. This means creating a space where you both feel comfortable being vulnerable and expressing your feelings without fear of judgment or rejection.

Practice active listening: Part of building trust involves listening actively to your partner. Listening requires understanding and responding with empathy. You should be present, focus on what your partner is saying, and validate their feelings.

Use "I" statements: You should be able to express your feelings and desires freely without placing blame or sounding accusatory. This means using "I" statements instead of "you" statements. For example, instead of saying, "You never satisfy me," you could say, "I feel unsatisfied sometimes, and I want to explore new things with you."

Set the mood: Create a romantic atmosphere before sharing deep emotions. Get comfortable, take your time, and try to connect with each other on an emotional level.

Be respectful: Remember to respect your partner's boundaries. If they're not ready to share their deepest emotions yet, don't push them.

Sharing deep emotions during sex is a top tip for couples to make sex more romantic and intimate because it entails creation of a stronger emotional bond between partners. It is easy to get lost in the physical sensations of sex and forget the emotional connection that exists between partners. Sharing deep emotions during sexual intimacy allows partners to open up to each other, leading to a deeper understanding and appreciation of each other's needs.

When done successfully, sharing deep emotions during sex can lead to better communication, trust, and intimacy in the relationship. By being vulnerable with your partner, you create a safe space that encourages them to do the same, opening up channels for honest conversations. It can also lead to meaningful discoveries about each other that deepen the bond between partners.

Moreover, discussing feelings and desires during intimacy helps partners explore new and exciting ways of experiencing pleasure together. By being open about what they want, couples can try out new things that bring them closer and make their sexual experiences more satisfying. It is hard to refuse putting your desires into action when your partner is fully committed to making you happy and satisfied. Expressing emotions during sex also helps partners feel more seen and heard, increasing their confidence and satisfaction in the relationship.

However, it's important to remember that sharing deep emotions during sex isn't for everyone. Both partners must be comfortable and willing to participate in this level of emotional intimacy. Some people may feel insecure or embarrassed to share their innermost feelings and desires during sexual activity. In such cases, it's best to communicate openly outside of an intimate sexual setting, and with time, you can build up enough trust to share deeper emotions during sex.

In conclusion, creating a safe space where both partners can express their deepest thoughts, desires, and feelings is crucial for building trust, improving communication, and ultimately improving intimacy within a sexual relationship. Remember to build trust, actively listen, use "I" statements, set the mood, and be respectful to your partner's boundaries in order to successfully share deep emotions during sex. This is a simple cheat sheet for couples to make sex more romantic and intimate, and it can lead to more meaningful, satisfying, and enjoyable sexual experiences that deepen the relationship.

So, if you want to take your sexual relationship with your partner to the next level, try incorporating the tip of sharing deep emotions during sex. It can be the key to experiencing a deeper emotional connection with your partner, better communication, and an overall more fulfilling relationship.

Chapter 7

Communicate Your Desires

Communication is so important in a romantic relationship. When it comes to sex, it's absolutely essential for both partners to feel safe and comfortable expressing what they want and need.

Here are some tips on how to communicate your desires:

Make time for conversation: It's important to set aside dedicated time to talk about your sexual desires without interruption or distraction.

Practice active listening: This means really listening to your partner's desires and needs without interrupting, being defensive, or passing judgment. Try to understand where they're coming from without feeling like you need to solve their problems.

Use "I" statements: Instead of saying "you never do this" or "you always do that," focus on how you feel and what you want. For example, "I would really love it if we could try X" or "I feel really loved when we do Y." This approach is less confrontational and more likely to lead to positive changes.

Be open-minded: Remember that everyone has different desires and fantasies. Be open to exploring new things with your partner, even if they are not something you've ever considered before.

Be honest and direct: Don't beat around the bush or use vague language when talking about your desires. Speak honestly and directly in a way that your partner can understand.

Check in regularly: Just like any other aspect of a relationship, sexual desires can change over time. Make sure to check in with your partner regularly to make sure you're both still on the same page.

By communicating your desires openly and honestly, you can create a safe, trusting, and intimate space for both partners to enjoy.

Communicating your desires is one of the top tips for couples to make sex more romantic and intimate because when both partners feel heard and validated, it creates a deeper sense of connection and intimacy between them. It also helps to build trust and understanding, which can make it easier to experiment with new things and try out different fantasies.

Simple Cheat Sheet for Romantic Sex

When you're able to talk about your desires without fear of judgment or rejection, it can also help to alleviate any anxieties or insecurities you may have about your own sexuality. This, in turn, can lead to a more relaxed and enjoyable sexual experience for both partners.

Ultimately, being open and honest about your desires can help to create a more satisfying, fulfilling sex life that brings you closer together as a couple.

By communicating your desires, you can also help to establish boundaries and create a sense of safety in your sexual relationship. This is especially important when it comes to trying out new things or exploring new fantasies. When both partners feel comfortable speaking up about what they do and don't want, it creates an atmosphere of trust and respect that can be essential for trying out new experiences.

In addition to helping to build intimacy and trust, communicating your desires can also lead to better sexual satisfaction. When both partners are aware of what the other person wants and needs, they can work together to find ways to satisfy each other more fully. This can lead to a more fulfilling sexual experience for both partners.

So, if you're looking to make sex more romantic and intimate with your partner, start by communicating your desires openly and honestly. By doing so, you can help to strengthen your bond with each other and create a more fulfilling and enjoyable sex life. Remember to be patient and understanding with each other, as it can take time to learn how to communicate effectively about sex. But with practice and open-mindedness, you can build a strong foundation of trust and intimacy that will help to make your sexual relationship more fulfilling and satisfying for years to come.

Simple Cheat Sheet for Romantic Sex

Chapter 8

Try New Things

Exploring new positions, techniques, and toys can be a fun and exciting way to keep things fresh and exciting in the bedroom.

Here are some tips on how to try new things:

Communicate with your partner: Before trying anything new, make sure to talk about it with your partner and get their input. Make sure you're both on the same page about what you want to try.

Be open-minded: Remember that trying something new doesn't mean you have to completely change your sexual identity. Be open to experimenting and exploring, but always stay true to your own boundaries and comfort levels.

Do your research: If you're interested in trying out a new position or technique, do your research ahead of time to make sure you know what you're doing. This can help to reduce awkwardness and uncertainty in the moment.

Start slowly: If you're new to exploring new positions, techniques, or toys, it's important to start slowly and work your way up. Begin with something simple and gradually build up to more complex acts.

Create a comfortable environment: Trying new things can be nerve-wracking, so make sure to create a comfortable and relaxed environment to help put you both at ease. This can include lighting candles, playing music, or even setting up some comfortable pillows.

Cheryl Bach

Experiment with toys: Sex toys can be a fun and exciting addition to your sexual relationship. Start with something simple, like a vibrator or a blindfold, and then add more complex toys as you become more comfortable.

Exploring new positions, techniques, and toys can be a great way to keep things fresh and exciting in the bedroom. It can help to break down barriers and create a deeper sense of intimacy and connection between you and your partner. This is why trying new things is one of the top tips for couples to make sex more romantic and intimate.

When you try out new positions, techniques or toys, it allows you to discover what turns your partner on and what really gets them going. It also helps to keep your sexual relationship from becoming stagnant or monotonous, which can happen over time if you stick to the same routine.

Simple Cheat Sheet for Romantic Sex

By trying new things, you can also gain a deeper understanding of your own desires and preferences. You might discover that you enjoy something that you never thought you would or that a new position makes you feel like a whole new person.

In addition to enhancing your physical connection, trying new things can also help to build trust and communication in your relationship. When you're both open to exploring new things together, it creates an atmosphere of trust and respect that can help to strengthen your bond and deepen your intimacy.

It's important to remember that trying new things doesn't have to be complicated or intimidating. It can be as simple as trying out a new position, incorporating some light bondage play, or experimenting with a new sex toy. The most important thing is to communicate openly with your partner and to prioritize each other's pleasure and comfort.

Overall, trying new things is a great way for couples to keep their sex life exciting, adventurous, and fulfilling. It helps you to discover new sides of yourself and your partner, and strengthens the emotional connection between you. So, don't be afraid to step outside your comfort zone and try something new - you just might be surprised by how much fun you have!

Simple Cheat Sheet for Romantic Sex

Chapter 9

Engage in Foreplay

Engaging in foreplay is one of the simplest and most effective ways to build anticipation and heighten the mood during sexual activity.

Here are some tips on how to go about it:

Take your time: The whole point of foreplay is to take your time and enjoy the build-up to sex. Don't rush into anything - take your time to kiss, touch, and explore each other's bodies.

Try different techniques: Foreplay isn't just about kissing and touching. There are plenty of different techniques you can try, such as massaging each other, using toys, or even watching porn together.

Communicate with your partner: Make sure to communicate with your partner about what turns you on and what feels good. This can help to create a deeper level of intimacy and trust between you.

Be generous: Make sure to give as much as you receive during foreplay. Don't just focus on your own pleasure, but also focus on satisfying and pleasing your partner.

Set the mood: Create a comfortable, romantic environment to help set the mood for foreplay. This can include lighting candles, playing soft music, or even having a glass of champagne.

Use your senses: Engage all of your senses during foreplay. Use touch, scent, taste, sight and sound to heighten the mood and build anticipation.

Be creative: Don't be afraid to get creative during foreplay. Try out new techniques and explore each other's bodies in different ways to keep things fresh and exciting.

Engaging in foreplay is one of the top tips for couples to make sex more romantic and intimate for a number of reasons. First, it helps to build anticipation and heighten the mood, which can make sex feel more exciting and fulfilling. Foreplay also allows you to explore each other's bodies and discover what turns each other on, which can help to strengthen your connection and deepen your intimacy.

Moreover, engaging in foreplay helps to create a slower and more deliberate approach to sex, which is often more romantic and intimate than rushing into sex without warming up first. By taking the time to build up arousal and excitement through foreplay, you're setting the stage for a more passionate and fulfilling experience. Foreplay is also an important way to connect emotionally with your partner before having sex. By communicating with your partner about what feels good and what you both want out of the experience, you're building trust and intimacy that can translate into a more satisfying sexual relationship.

Overall, engaging in foreplay is a crucial ingredient for making sex more romantic and intimate for couples. It helps to create a sense of intimacy and closeness while also building anticipation and excitement. By taking the time to explore each other's bodies and desires, you're creating a deeper level of trust and communication that will only enhance your sexual experiences.

In addition, incorporating more foreplay into your sexual routine can actually improve the physical aspects of your sexual encounters. By taking your time to warm up and build arousal, the end result is often more intense orgasms and a more satisfying experience overall.

But it's important to note that foreplay isn't just about physical pleasure - it's also about emotional connection. By engaging in intimate touching, kissing and caressing, you're creating a deeper bond that can translate into a more fulfilling relationship outside of the bedroom.

So whether you're in a long-term relationship or just starting out with a new partner, taking the time to engage in foreplay is a crucial component of making sex more romantic and intimate. It's all about taking your time, communicating with your partner, and exploring each other's bodies and desires. By incorporating more foreplay into your sexual routine, you can create a deeper sense of connection and intimacy that will only enhance your overall relationship.

Simple Cheat Sheet for Romantic Sex

To make the most of your foreplay experience, communication is key. Make sure to talk openly with your partner about what feels good, what you want to try, and what makes you both feel comfortable. Take your time to explore each other's bodies and desires, trying out different techniques and finding out what works best for you both.

Overall, engaging in foreplay is an essential part of making sex more romantic and intimate. By building anticipation, exploring each other's desires, and connecting emotionally and physically, you can create meaningful and satisfying sexual experiences that deepen your bond with your partner. Remember to take it slow, communicate openly, and have fun exploring each other's bodies and desires. With these tips, you can easily incorporate more foreplay into your sexual routine and reap the benefits of a more romantic and intimate sexual relationship.

Chapter 10

Make Eye Contact

Maintaining eye contact during sex is an often-overlooked but incredibly powerful way to deepen intimacy and heighten the romantic connection between you and your partner. Eye contact can allow couples to communicate on a deeper level and create an emotional bond that makes the physical experience more fulfilling and satisfying.

So, how exactly do you go about making eye contact during sex? Here are some simple tips to help you get started:

Start slow: It can be intimidating to lock eyes with your partner during sex, especially if you're not used to it. So, start slowly by maintaining eye contact during moments of intimacy that feel comfortable and natural.

Use foreplay as a warm-up: Engage in eye contact during foreplay as a way to build anticipation and heighten the mood. Make eye contact while kissing, touching, or caressing your partner to create a deeper sense of intimacy and connection. This can also help you both to feel more comfortable and relaxed during sex, making it easier to maintain eye contact.

Focus on your partner's eyes: When you're locking eyes with your partner, try to focus on their eyes and the emotions you see there. This can help you to stay present in the moment and appreciate the beauty of your partner, as well as deepen your emotional connection.

Try different positions: Experiment with different sexual positions that allow for eye contact, such as missionary, cowgirl, or spooning. This can add an extra layer of intimacy and make the experience even more romantic and satisfying.

Communicate with your eyes: Eye contact can also be a powerful way to communicate with your partner during sex. Use your eyes to express your desires, communicate when something feels good, and show your partner how much you care. This can be especially helpful for couples who have trouble communicating verbally about their sexual needs.

Making eye contact during sex is one of the top tips for couples to make sex more romantic and intimate because it deepens emotional connection and creates a sense of vulnerability between partners. Eye contact can help couples to feel more connected, present, and engaged in the moment. It can also create a deeper bond that extends beyond the physical and into the emotional realm.

Moreover, eye contact during sex can help to build trust and intimacy between partners. When you're locking eyes with your partner, you're showing them that you trust them, that you're vulnerable with them, and that you care deeply about them. This can strengthen the emotional connection between partners, leading to a more satisfying and fulfilling relationship both in and outside of the bedroom.

In conclusion, making eye contact during sex is a simple yet powerful way to deepen intimacy and create a more meaningful sexual experience with your partner. It can help to enhance emotional connection, build trust, and heighten the romantic bond between partners. With these tips, you can begin to incorporate eye contact into your sexual routine and reap the benefits of a more intimate and fulfilling sexual relationship with your partner.

Chapter 11

Cuddle and Hold Each Other After

The intimacy of sex doesn't have to end after orgasm. Couples can cnhance the emotional connection between them by continuing to cuddle and hold each other after sex. Simply lying together in each other's arms can create a warm and comforting environment that extends the romantic bond beyond the physical moment.

So, how do you go about cuddling and holding each other after sex?

Take your time: Don't rush to get up and leave the bed after sex. Spend some time cuddling, holding each other or simply lying together in silence. This can allow you both to bask in the afterglow of the experience and deepen your emotional connection.

Communicate: While you're lying in each other's arms, take the time to communicate with each other about how you're feeling and what you enjoyed about the experience. This can help to build an even deeper emotional bond between partners and make the experience even more romantic and intimate.

Practice touch: Use this time to intimately explore each other's bodies through touch. Gently running your fingers over your partner's skin can create a sense of intimacy and comfort that extends beyond the physical act of sex.

Embrace the silence: Sometimes, the most intimate moments are the ones shared in silence. Enjoy the quiet moments snuggled up in each other's arms and let the intimacy speak for itself.

Cuddling and holding each other after sex is one of the top tips for couples to make sex more romantic and intimate because it not only adds an extra layer of physical intimacy but also emotional intimacy. It allows couples to spend time bonding and connecting on a deeper level, which can make the sexual experience even more meaningful and satisfying.

When you cuddle and hold each other after sex, you're creating a space for vulnerability and intimacy between partners. It's a way to show your partner that you're comfortable and safe with them, and it can help couples to build trust and strengthen their emotional connection.

Additionally, cuddling and holding each other after sex can have physical health benefits as well. It can lower stress and anxiety levels in both partners, reducing the risk of heart disease and other health issues.

Simple Cheat Sheet for Romantic Sex

In conclusion, taking the time to cuddle and hold each other after sex is a simple yet effective way to add comfort and connection to your intimacy. It allows couples to deepen their emotional bond and create a safe and loving space for each other. So, next time you engage in sex with your partner, take the time to snuggle up close and hold each other, and enjoy the intimate moment of connection that it brings. Remember, intimacy doesn't have to end after orgasm, and by following this simple tip, you can make your sexual experiences more romantic and satisfying than ever before.

Furthermore, it's important to note that cuddling and holding each other after sex is not just limited to heterosexual relationships, as everyone can enjoy the benefits of this intimate experience. All couples, no matter what their sexual orientation is, can take advantage of this simple yet powerful tip to deepen their romantic and emotional connection.

In summary, the beauty of cuddling and holding each other after sex is that it's a simple, yet effective way to add comfort and connection to your intimacy. It's a way for couples to deepen their bond and create a nurturing and safe environment for each other. Incorporating this tip into your sexual routine can bring a new level of intimacy and emotional connection to your relationship.

So go ahead, take your time after sex, communicate with your partner, explore touch, and embrace the silence. Just remember that the most important thing is to enjoy each other's company and create a space of comfort and connection.

In conclusion, cuddling and holding each other after sex is one of the simplest yet most effective tips for couples to make sex more romantic and intimate. Whether you're starting a new relationship or have been with your partner for years, taking the time to snuggle up close and enjoy

Simple Cheat Sheet for Romantic Sex

each other's company can deepen your emotional bond and create an even more meaningful sexual experience.

Chapter 12

Share Fantasies

Sharing your sexual fantasies with your partner is a powerful way to deepen the intimacy in your relationship. It allows you to explore your desires and create a safe and open space for both partners to express themselves without fear of judgment or rejection. When done correctly, sharing your fantasies can lead to more fulfilling, romantic, and intimate sexual experiences.

So, how do you go about sharing your fantasies with your partner?

Trust and Communication: The first step in sharing your sexual fantasies is building trust and open communication with your partner. It's important to feel comfortable with each other and be able to share your deepest desires without fear of judgment.

Start Small: You don't have to go all-in when sharing your fantasies with your partner. Start with something small to get the conversation going and build from there. This can be something as simple as a new position or talking about trying a new role-play scenario. As you become more comfortable sharing your desires, you can continue to build on these conversations and explore more complex fantasies.

Timing: Timing is everything when it comes to sharing your sexual fantasies. Make sure that your partner is receptive and open to having this conversation, and that you're both in a relaxed and comfortable state of mind. Avoid bringing up these types of conversations during stressful or tense moments, as it can lead to miscommunication or misunderstandings.

Be Respectful: It's important to be respectful of your partner's boundaries when sharing your fantasies. If your partner is not comfortable with a certain scenario or idea, it's important to respect their wishes and not push the issue. Conversely, if your partner shares a fantasy with you that you're not comfortable with, communicate your boundaries in a respectful and understanding way.

Mutual exploration: Sharing your fantasies is not a one-sided activity, it's important to explore your partner's fantasies as well. Engage in mutual exploration, where both partners can share their desires and fantasies and respectfully discuss ways to make them a reality.

Why is Sharing Fantasies a Top Tip for Couples to Make Sex More Romantic and Intimate?

Sharing your sexual fantasies with your partner is a powerful way to build intimacy and improve your sexual relationship. It allows you to explore your desires together and communicate openly about what works and what doesn't. By sharing fantasies, you are creating a safe and open space for both partners to express themselves without fear of judgment or rejection. This positive sharing of mutual desires can lead to more romantic and intimate sexual experiences that are tailored to the desires of both partners.

Additionally, sharing your fantasies can also bring a sense of excitement and novelty to your sexual relationship. It allows you and your partner to explore new experiences and scenarios, which can help keep the passion alive in your relationship. By sharing your fantasies, you are creating a deeper and more meaningful connection with your partner that can help increase intimacy and strengthen your bond.

Finally, sharing your fantasies can help build trust and encourage communication in your relationship. By being open and honest about your desires, you are telling your partner that you trust them enough to share these intimate thoughts with them. This increased level of trust and communication can lead to a stronger and more fulfilling relationship both inside and outside of the bedroom.

In conclusion, sharing your sexual fantasies with your partner is a top tip for couples to make sex more romantic and intimate because it encourages exploration, creates excitement, and improves communication and trust in the relationship. It's important to approach these conversations with respect, trust, and an open mind to create a safe space for both partners to express themselves. Ultimately, sharing your fantasies can lead to a more fulfilling and satisfying sexual relationship where both partners feel heard and understood. So why not take the plunge and start exploring your desires together? You might be surprised at what you discover.

Simple Cheat Sheet for Romantic Sex

Chapter 13

Practice Gratitude

Expressing gratitude to your partner before, during, and after sexual experiences can increase the romantic and intimate connection between couples. Gratitude is the act of appreciating what we have in our lives, including the love, commitment, and trust that our partners bring to our sexual relationships. By practicing gratitude, couples can create a positive and fulfilling sexual experience while also improving their overall relationship.

So, how do you go about practicing gratitude with your partner during sexual experiences?

Verbal Communication: Verbal communication is key when it comes to expressing gratitude during sex. Use words of affirmation like "thank you," or "I appreciate you" throughout the experience. Validate your partner's feelings by letting them know how much you appreciate their trust, love, and commitment.

Non-Verbal Communication: Non-verbal communication can also play a big role in expressing gratitude during sex. Use your body language to convey appreciation, such as holding your partner tightly or caressing their body. Make eye contact and smile to let your partner know how much you enjoy being intimate with them.

Touching: Touch is a key component of sexual intimacy, but it can also be used to express gratitude. Use touch to communicate your gratitude during sex, whether it's holding hands, embracing, or stroking your partner's face. Physical touch is a powerful way to show your partner how much you appreciate them and the bond you share.

Gifts: Surprising your partner with a small gift before or after sex can also express gratitude. It doesn't have to be extravagant or expensive, but something simple like a love note or a favorite treat can show your partner that you are thinking of them and appreciate them.

Acknowledge the effort: Acknowledge the effort your partner puts into building and maintaining an intimate, romantic relationship. Recognize the little things that they do, such as planning a special date or setting the mood for a romantic evening.

Why is Practicing Gratitude a Top Tip for Couples to Make Sex More Romantic and Intimate?

Being grateful for your partner and expressing appreciation during sexual experiences can increase the romantic and intimate connection between couples. Gratitude promotes positive feelings and can help combat negative emotions like anxiety or stress that might interfere with intimacy.

Simple Cheat Sheet for Romantic Sex

When we experience gratitude, it increases our sense of well-being and deepens the connection we feel to our partners.

Moreover, practicing gratitude during sex can also increase feelings of trust and commitment between partners. When we take time to express our appreciation, it reinforces the bond we share with our partners and strengthens the trust and commitment we have to each other. By being grateful for our partner's love, trust, and commitment, we show them that we value and respect the relationship we share.

Additionally, expressing gratitude during sex can also promote a positive and fulfilling sexual experience. By acknowledging the effort our partners put into the relationship, we increase their sense of self-worth and make them feel valued. This positive reinforcement in turn helps create a mutually satisfying sexual experience.

In conclusion, practicing gratitude during sexual experiences is an important way to deepen the connection between partners and increase feelings of trust, commitment, and intimacy. It promotes positive emotions and helps create a positive and fulfilling sexual experience. By expressing appreciation for our partner's love, trust, and commitment, we strengthen the bond we share and deepen the romantic and intimate connection between couples.

Simple Cheat Sheet for Romantic Sex

Chapter 14

Don't Neglect Non-Sexual Touch

When we think about intimacy in a sexual context, physical touch is often the first thing that comes to mind. However, non-sexual touch plays a crucial role in building and maintaining feelings of love and intimacy between partners. In this chapter, we will explore the importance of non-sexual touch and provide tips on how couples can engage in it to build a stronger, more intimate relationship.

Why Don't Neglect Non-Sexual Touch is a Top Tip for Couples to Make Sex More Romantic and Intimate?

Non-sexual touch is essential because it builds feelings of love and intimacy outside of the bedroom and helps promote a deeper connection between couples. Research suggests that regular, affectionate touch – whether kissing, hugging, holding hands, or stroking - can have significant mental and physical health benefits for both partners in a relationship. In fact, studies have shown that non-sexual touch can reduce stress hormones, increase feelings of well-being, and promote feelings of closeness and attachment between partners.

By engaging in non-sexual touch throughout the day, couples can deepen their emotional connection and create a more romantic and intimate environment. This, in turn, can lead to more satisfying sexual experiences in the bedroom as partners are more open and vulnerable with each other.

How to Incorporate Non-Sexual Touch into Your Daily Routine?

The first step in incorporating non-sexual touch into your daily routine is to start small. Begin by hugging or kissing each other when you say goodbye or hello or holding hands while hanging out together. You can also try giving your partner a shoulder massage after a long day at work or stroking their hair when they are feeling stressed. The idea is to create opportunities for physical affection that are not necessarily sexual in nature.

Another way to engage in non-sexual touch is by engaging in activities together that involve physical touch. For example, taking a dance class together, going on a hike and holding hands, or even cooking a meal together and brushing up against each other in the kitchen can create opportunities for non-sexual touch.

It's important to be mindful of your partner's comfort level and boundaries when engaging in non-sexual touch. Communicate openly with each other and ask for consent before touching or engaging in physical activities together. If either partner feels uncomfortable or overwhelmed, it's important to respect their boundaries and find alternative ways to build intimacy.

In conclusion, incorporating non-sexual touch into your daily routine may seem like a small action, but it can have a significant impact on your relationship. It helps promote feelings of love and intimacy, reduces stress, and creates a stronger emotional connection between partners. By engaging in non-sexual touch throughout your day, you can create a more romantic and intimate environment and ultimately lead to more satisfying sexual experiences with your partner.

Remember that physical touch is just one aspect of building a strong and healthy relationship, and it's important to also make time for emotional intimacy and communication. By prioritizing both physical and emotional intimacy, you can create a better-rounded and fulfilling relationship with your partner.

So, take the time to hug, kiss, and hold hands with your partner throughout the day. Be mindful of each other's comfort levels and boundaries, and communicate openly to ensure that both partners are feeling safe and comfortable. These small acts of non-sexual touch can go a long way in building a more loving and intimate relationship.

Simple Cheat Sheet for Romantic Sex

Chapter 15

Be Open and Vulnerable

Sex is not just about physical sensations; it's also about emotional connection. Being open and vulnerable with your partner is essential to building intimacy and increasing feelings of connection during a sexual experience. In this chapter, we will explore why being open and vulnerable is important in building a romantic sexual experience and provide tips on how couples can go about it.

Why Being Open and Vulnerable is a Top Tip for Couples to Make Sex More Romantic and Intimate?

Sex is more than just a physical act; it's an emotional and mental experience too. By being open and vulnerable, partners can create a deeper emotional connection and build trust with each other. This can lead to an increased sense of closeness and intimacy, which can ultimately lead to more satisfying sexual experiences.

When partners are open and vulnerable with each other, they are showing their true selves and allowing themselves to be seen in a raw and authentic way. This level of vulnerability can be scary, but it can also be liberating and empowering. It can help partners feel more connected to each other and create a sense of safety and trust in the experience.

Furthermore, being open and vulnerable during sex can help partners communicate their desires and needs more effectively. By being honest and candid with each other, partners can ensure that both parties are feeling heard and satisfied in the sexual experience. This can lead to a more fulfilling and satisfying sexual encounter for both partners.

Cheryl Bach

Tips on Being Open and Vulnerable During a Romantic Sexual Experience

Practice Communication: Communication is key when it comes to being open and vulnerable during sex. Help build emotional intimacy by talking about your feelings and desires before, during, and after the sexual experience.

Trust Your Partner: Trust is an essential component of being open and vulnerable during sex. Make sure to build trust with your partner by creating a safe space where both parties feel comfortable expressing themselves.

Take Your Time: Being open and vulnerable can be difficult, so make sure to take your time and move at a pace that feels comfortable for both partners. Don't rush or push yourself – allow yourself to fully relax and be present in the experience.

Be Willing to Experiment: Being open and vulnerable means being willing to try new things together. Experimenting with different techniques and positions can help partners feel more connected and build a deeper sense of intimacy.

Focus on Pleasure: When couples focus on pleasure rather than performing, they are more likely to let their guard down and be vulnerable. Make sure to prioritize pleasure and enjoy the experience together.

Learn to Read Each Other's Cues: Being attuned to each other's nonverbal cues can help partners feel more connected and build a deeper sense of intimacy. Pay attention to your partner's body language and respond accordingly.

Practice Mindfulness: Being present and in the moment during sex can help partners feel more connected emotionally and physically. Practice mindfulness by focusing on your breath and staying present in your body and in the experience.

Avoid Judgment: Being open and vulnerable requires a judgment-free space. Avoid judging yourself or your partner, and instead focus on creating a positive and supportive environment.

Share Your Fantasies: Sharing your fantasies with your partner can help build intimacy and trust. Be open and honest about what you desire and allow your partner to do the same.

Be Genuine: Being open and vulnerable means being true to yourself and your feelings. Don't pretend to feel a certain way or try to please your partner – instead, be authentic and true to yourself.

Simple Cheat Sheet for Romantic Sex

Embrace Imperfection: Being vulnerable means embracing imperfection and being okay with making mistakes. Remember that it's okay to be imperfect and that it's all part of the process of building intimacy and trust with your partner.

Take Time for Aftercare: Aftercare is an important part of being open and vulnerable during a romantic sexual experience. Make sure to take time to cuddle, talk, and connect with your partner after the experience to help build emotional intimacy and foster a sense of closeness.

In conclusion, being open and vulnerable is a crucial component of building a romantic and intimate sexual experience. By practicing good communication, building trust, and staying present in the moment, couples can deepen their emotional connection and create more satisfying sexual experiences. By being genuine and authentic, partners can create a judgment-free space that allows for exploration and experimentation. Remember to embrace imperfection and take time for aftercare to foster emotional connection and build intimacy with your partner. By incorporating these tips into your sexual experiences, you can make sex more than just a physical act and create a deeper sense of intimacy and connection with your partner.

Simple Cheat Sheet for Romantic Sex

Conclusion

To wrap up our journey into the world of romantic and intimate sex, let us consider all that we have learned in Simple Cheat Sheet for Romantic Sex: 15 Tips for Couples to Make Sex More Romantic and Intimate.

We began by acknowledging how important it is to focus on each other, to remove any distractions, and create an atmosphere that encourages intimacy. Following these proven tips enhances the experience for both you and your partner. Then, as we progressed through the book, we looked at several ways in which communication and safety are central to romantic sexual encounters.

We explored the power of foreplay, engaging all senses, and taking things slow. We also discussed the power of physical touch, both inside and outside of the bedroom, as well as taking the time to connect emotionally and sharing your desires.

In addition, we talked about the importance of trying new things, exploring fantasies, and practicing gratitude. While it's important to embrace adventurousness in sex, it's equally important to maintain open communication with your partner about their desires and boundaries.

We have learned that creating a more romantic and intimate sexual experience is not just about physical touch and exploration. It's about creating a connection with your partner that goes beyond the surface level. This connection can be fostered through sharing of emotions during sex, expressing gratitude, and even cuddling after orgasm.

Mastering these 15 tips takes time and is an ongoing process of learning and communication. But with practice and patience, you and your partner can cultivate a more connected, loving, and fulfilling sexual relationship.

In conclusion, Simple Cheat Sheet for Romantic Sex: 15 Tips for Couples to Make Sex More Romantic and Intimate elucidates the power of understanding and meeting your partner's needs. With the tips shared in this book, you can transform your sexual relationship with your partner by deepening the bond between the two of you. Go forth and explore the possibilities of romance in sex. Create an ambiance that enhances intimacy, engage all senses, increase emotional connection, and experiment with new things. Remember, every relationship is unique, so find what works for you and your partner. By incorporating these tips into your sexual encounters, you can become a better partner, lover, and friend. Enjoy the journey toward a more fulfilling sexual relationship!

Simple Cheat Sheet for Romantic Sex

www.ingramcontent.com/pod-product-compliance
Lightning Source LLC
Chambersburg PA
CBHW050814250726

48653CB00006B/2223